Fiber Foods: Use Natural Fiber, Bran, soluble fiber, insoluble fiber to Propel Your Health Upward

"Change your Life, Eliminate Disease with Fiber"
The Nutritional Series: Volume 1

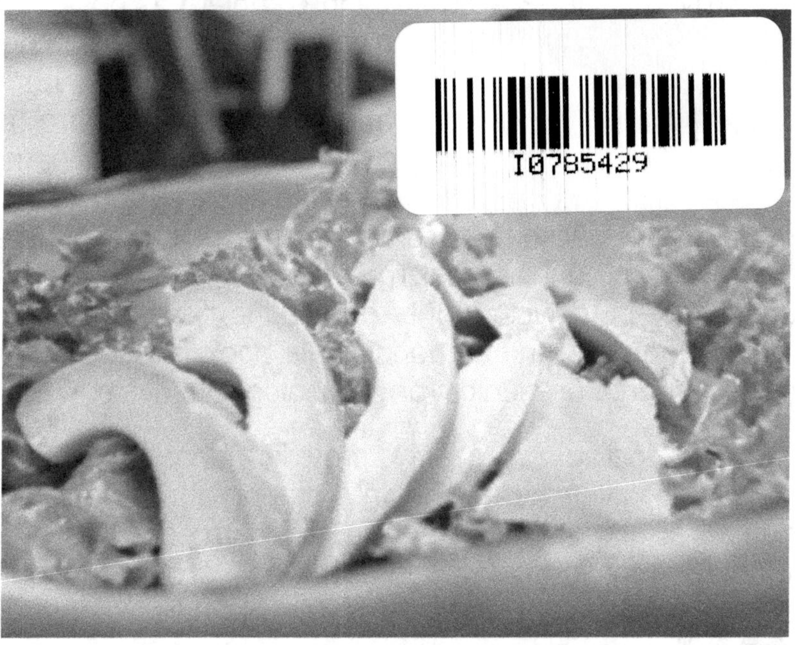

By Rudy S Silva, Nutritional Consultant

Disclaimer and Terms of Use: The Author and Publisher have strived to be as accurate and complete as possible in the creation of this book, notwithstanding the fact that he does not warrant or represent at any time that the contents within are accurate due to the rapidly changing nature of the Internet and nutritional science. While all attempts have been made to verify information provided in this publication, the Author and Publisher assume no responsibility for errors, omissions, or contrary interpretation of the subject matter herein. Any perceived slights of specific persons, peoples, or organizations are unintentional. This book is not intended for use as a source of medical or psychological advice.

Your doctor or health provider should confirm any information given here. This information should not be taken as medical or psychiatric advice or treatment. This e-book is for information and educational purposes only. Consult with your doctor before using any of the remedies or information listed in the e-book.

Printed in the United States of America

Table of Contents

1: Introduction to Fiber Foods

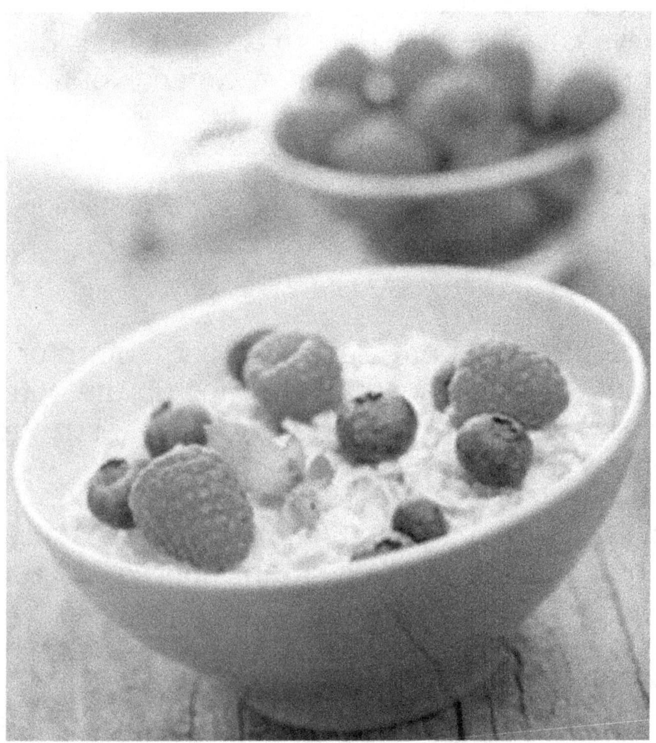

This is a new series on nutritional health. This book is a no-nonsense approach with to the point information on fiber. It will give you quick information on fiber. You can, then, start using and applying the ideas presented right away. After reading this book, you will be able to immediately add more foods to your menu that will provide you with the fiber you need.

Fiber has its own high-level position in nutrition. It is a critical element necessary for creating the best health possible. Most people concentrate on vitamins, minerals, fats, carbohydrates, and protein to create a healthy menu. They don't always consider that they must have near 35 grams of fiber every day to ensure the proper workings of their body.

So, let's get right to it, and discover the true importance of fiber. Discover what you need to do to get more of this nutrient into your body.

What is Fiber?

Fiber comes only from plants and is the form or structure of that plant. It is that part that makes up the outer cellular structure of the plant. Fiber gives form and strength to **fruits, vegetables, and grains**.

Fiber is called by many names – bulk, roughage, or dietary fiber, but the most important fiber is call soluble and insoluble fiber.

Fiber consists of many different chemical substances and forms. It can be hard, rigid, soft, and gummy. The hard fiber is called insoluble cellulose found mostly in vegetables and grains. The soft fiber is called soluble fiber, which is found in fruits and vegetables.

Fiber is a non-starch polysaccharide, which is called cellulose, dextrin, inulin, lignin, chitins, pectin, beta-glycan, waxes, and oligosaccharides.

Two Types of Fiber – Soluble, Insoluble

Soluble fiber dissolves in water, which passes easily into the small intestine. In the small and large intestine, it is fermented by bacteria. With water, soluble fiber turns gelatinous. It is fermented by bacteria as it goes through the small and large intestines.

Insoluble fiber does not dissolve in water. As it goes through the digestive tract, it does not change its form.

To reach a high level of health, you need to eat both soluble and insoluble fibers.

Dietary fiber foods are generally divided into predominantly soluble or insoluble. Both types of fiber are present in all plant foods, but rarely in equal proportions.

Most of the soluble fiber, in fruits, should be eaten in the morning. This fiber digests faster, which helps to detoxify your body. Insoluble fiber, in vegetables, should be eaten during lunch and dinner. They combine with your protein and carbohydrates to form stools that move quickly through your colon. Stools that remain too long in your colon produce toxins that get into your blood.

When fiber enters the stomach, stomach acid and digestive enzymes cannot break it down. This fiber remains in tack until it reaches the colon. There in the colon, fiber is partially digested by the good bacteria allowing the good bacteria to multiply, which makes you healthier. When you don't eat enough fiber, the good bacteria diminish and the bad bacteria multiply

Where to Get More Fiber

When you add more fiber to your diet, I'm not talking about the fiber you can find in a cereal box or fiber products at your drug store. I'm talking fiber in fruits, vegetables, seeds, and nuts.

If you use pure box fiber or other fiber products that guarantee constipation results, you run the risk of damaging the function of your colon. Box fiber and other drugstore fiber remedies can become addictive. The result can be that you cannot have a bowel movement without them. Artificial fiber does not have the nutrients, vitamins, and minerals in the balance you need for rebuilding and normalizing your colon.

35 Grams of Fiber Everyday

Your body needs between 35 to 45 gm. of fiber every day. Start adding more fiber to your diet, and eventually, you will be eating up to 35 grams, without knowing it. If you are like most people, you are only getting 8 grams of fiber every day, a recipe for poor long-term health.

If you are not used to consuming a lot of fiber, when you start eating more, initially, you will have some side effects, such as bloating, burping, or flatulence. These effects will disappear in 2—3 weeks as your body gets used to increased fiber. The good aspect of more fiber is you will have more bowel movements.

For good health, you should have at least two bowel movements per day; one in the morning and one after lunch or dinner. The ideal case is to have three bowel movements per day if you eat three meals per day.

If you don't have a bowel movement every day, then, you are constipated. There will be days when you don't have a bowel movement, but this should not be the norm.

2: How Fiber Helps Prevent Constipation

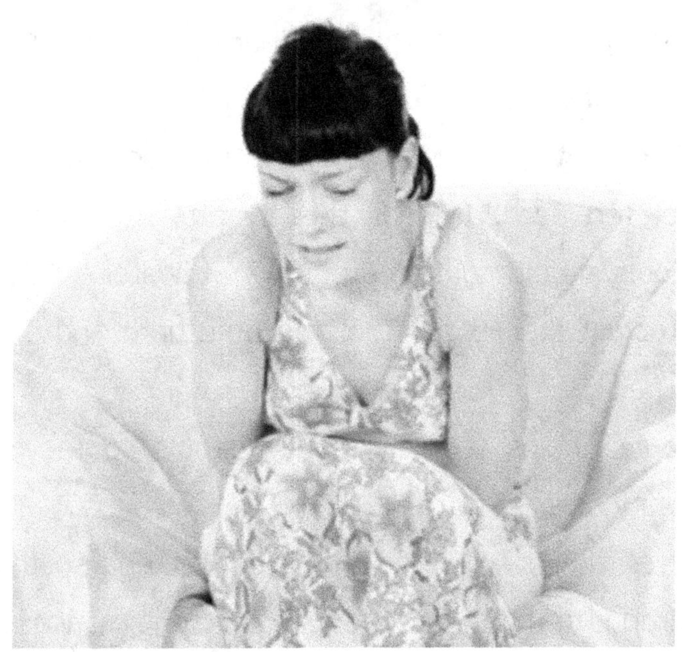

Enzymes and Fiber

Your body does not have the enzymes to break down fiber. So it enters your body in food and leaves it with very little change. It is during its travel down your gastrointestinal tract that it provides you with hundreds of benefits.

Fiber Benefits

As fiber enters the colon, here is how it helps to give you a daily bowel movement.

- One - scraps against your colon walls to keep it clean so that no sticky fecal matter buildup occurs there.

- Two - stimulates your colon walls to produce peristaltic movement that moves your fecal matter out your rectum. Without good peristaltic action, you will have constipation. The more fiber you eat the more peristaltic action you will experience.

- Three - it keeps moisture in your stools so they don't get too hard. It does this by attracting water. Your stools should contain around 75% water. Without the proper water level, stools become hard and difficult to expel.

- Four - helps you form bulky stools so they are not runny or extra hard.

- Five - helps you feed the good bacteria so they keep strong to fight off the bad bacteria. Once the bad bacteria take over, for sure you will have constipation.

- Six - helps to trap cholesterol, fats, toxins and excess estrogen and routes them out of your body. This prevents them from getting reabsorbed into your blood, causing health problems.

- Seven - Makes you feel fuller after a meal. Helps to control your appetite.

- Eight - Slows down the absorption of sugars and simple and complex carbohydrates, by holding them in the fiber matrix.

- Nine - Helps prevent colon cancer and other colon diseases, by moving toxic stools quickly out of your body.
- Ten – Helps in the control of diabetes, reduction of heart issues, and elimination of constipation, which prevents the formation of other diseases.

It is fiber that triggers the sensation of a pending bowel movement. It is fiber that helps you move your stool out of your body quickly. You should only take about 3-4 minutes to have a bowel movement. There should be no huffing or puffing to push out a stool. It should come out quickly and smoothly.

Two Bowel Movements Each Day

"If you don't have one bowel movement each day, you are constipated."

When you don't have one or two bowel movement per day, your fecal matter or stools remain in your colon longer than they should. This fecal matter is toxic and starts to produce gases and liquid that can flow through your colon walls and into your blood. Once in the blood, this toxicity moves throughout your body degrading cells, tissue, muscles, and organs. This toxicity can also enter your brain, which affects all brain functions.

Fiber Prevents Disease

There are many other health benefits when you consume the right amount of fiber. Fiber is important in the prevention or control of obesity, heart disease, diabetes, cancer, and colon diseases. If you have one of these diseases, consult with your doctor about increasing your fiber intake. If you have diverticulitis or colitis, definitely get your doctors opinion on eating more fiber.

"The deficiency of fiber in your diet should not be taken lightly."

Here is a list of some diseases or conditions that are related to the lack of fiber.

- Diabetes
- Gallstones
- Hemorrhoids
- Varicose veins
- Atherosclerosis
- Appendicitis
- Colitis
- Diverticulitis
- Colon cancer
- Deep Vein Thrombosis
- Increase Dental Cavities
- Constipation

3: The Best Time to Eat Fiber

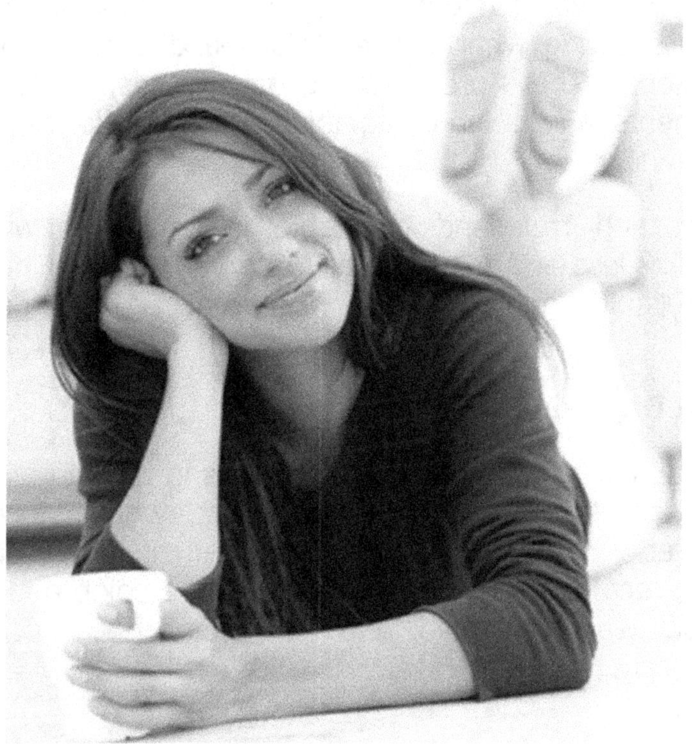

When to Eat Fruits

Now, when is the best time to eat fruits and vegetables? Here is one secret you may not hear elsewhere.

Eating fruits in the morning as solid fruits or in smoothies will help you detoxify. Fruits do this by pulling out toxins from your lymph liquid and blood that have accumulated there during the night.

Body's Detoxifying Cycle

Eat fruits, vegetables, fruits juices, vegetable juices, and water, between 8 am to noontime. In the morning until noon, your body is in a detoxification cycle. You can help this cycle by always eating what pushes this detoxification process to completion. The process needs liquids, fiber, and supplements. Fruits and vegetables contain up to 70-75% distilled water.

Fruit and fruit and vegetable juices digest within 90 minutes or less and move quickly into your colon. There they provide liquid, nutrients, and fiber that activate peristaltic action.

Protein Digestion

If you eat protein and carbohydrates in the morning, they take up to 4 hours or more to digest, which blocks your detoxification process. When the detoxifying process is blocked, fecal matter will accumulate in the colon and doesn't come out when it should. And, your colon does not cleanse out properly.

4: List-Best Fiber Foods to Eat

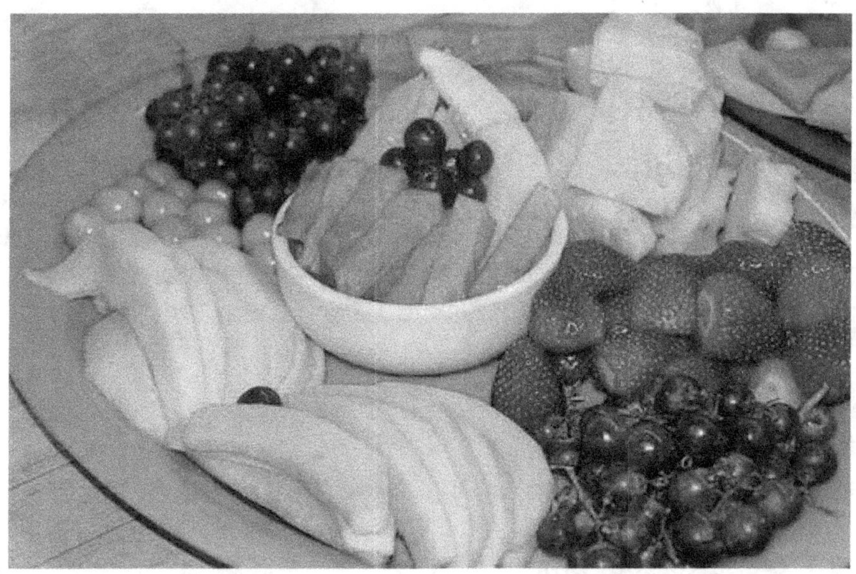

Fiber in Vegetables

All fruits and vegetables have some fiber. And, there are different types of fiber and each type has its health benefit. But, because you can get a good balance of these different fibers by eating a variety of the best fiber foods, there is no need to worry about what particular fiber you are eating.

Here is a way to get started getting more fiber into your diet. Start by eating more whole fruits or fruits in smoothies. Drink vegetable juices in the morning. If you are not able to juice vegetable, eat whole vegetables during lunch and dinner. Lightly cook vegetables to maintain the full properties of the fiber.

Add dried fruit to your diet, since it has higher fiber content. Dried fruit such as raisin, prunes, apricots, or apples can be eaten as snacks during your daily breaks. On occasion, eat seeds and nuts of various kinds as snacks or add them to your smoothies or salads.

Organic Produce

When you eat fruit leave the peel on, if it is organic. You can also leave the peel on potatoes and cucumbers. Most cucumbers have wax unless you buy them at the farmers market.

Bran Types

Add around 1 tablespoon of oat bran, rice bran, or chia seeds to your smoothies. You can experiment with how much bran to add to your smoothies.

Don't eat plain bran of any kind without drinking plenty of water afterward. Otherwise, it can become stuck in your colon without water.

Keep in mind that the laxative effects of various fiber foods will affect people differently. So, it is up to you to experiment with fiber foods to see which ones make you feel better.

Here is a list of the best fiber foods to eat.

The fiber foods listed at the top have the most fiber. Your challenge is to eat these fiber foods in the morning, lunch, and dinner so that you can get up to 35 grams. You can also eat some of them as snacks.

Eat fruits throughout the day, but especially in the evening. This will help to promote bowel movements in the morning. These are the fruits you should eat.

Food Chart Numbers

The following chart has food portions for specific foods and their fiber content. The fiber content numbers will vary based on the location where these fruits and vegetables were grown. These fiber numbers will give you a basic idea of which foods have more fiber.

The fiber numbers were not meant to be exact scientific numbers. Some of the foods listed do not have a portion listed. But, you can best guess that the portion will be ½ or 1 cup portions.

Use this chart to help you determine how much fiber you eat every day.

Fiber Chart

Food	Portion	Fiber (gm)
Beans black, cooked	1 cup	19.4
Kidney beans cooked	1 cup	19.4
Pinto beans canned or cooked	1 cup	18.8
Flour Masaharina (for tortillas)	1 cup	17
Baked beans in sauce (8-oz can)	1 cup	16
Baked beans with pork & molasses	1 cup	16

Rye flour (dark, whole grain)	1 cup	14.4
Flour Whole Wheat	1 cup	14.4
Peach dried, raw	1 large	14.3
Peas and carrots cooked	1 cup	13.4
Chickpeas (garbanzos) cooked	1 cup	12
Peas and carrots raw	1 cup	11.9
Kellogg's ® All-Bran Bran Buds	1/3 cup	11
Figs dried	3	10.5
Cereal All-Bran	1/2 cup	10.4
Cereal Bran Buds	1/2 cup	10.4
Figs stewed without sugar	3	10.3
Kellogg's® All-Bran (original)	½ cup	10
Kidney beans canned	1/2 cup	9.7
Figs stewed with sugar	3	9.7
Buckwheat grouts (kasha) cooked	1 cup	9.6
Bulgur, soaked cooked	1 cup	9.6
Peas green, fresh or frozen	1/2 cup	9.1
Currants, black raw		8.7
Horseradish, raw		8.3

Peanuts fresh		8.1
Peanuts roasted and salted		8.1
Prunes stewed without sugar	10	8.1
White beans canned or cooked	1/2 cup	8
most cereals	1 cup	8
black-eyed peas frozen/canned	1/2 cup	8
Raspberries	1 cup	8
Pinto beans	½ cup	8
Raspberries, stewed without sugar	1/2 cup	7.8
Cereal oatmeal	3/4 cup	7.7
Prunes stewed with sugar	10	7.7
Peanut butter smooth		7.6
Currants, black stewed without sugar		7.4
Raspberries, raw	1/2 cup	7.4
Beans baked, canned in tomato sauce		7.3
Bread high-bran "health" bread	2 slices	7
Broccoli fresh, cooked	3/4 cup	7
Raspberries, stewed with sugar	1/2 cup	7
Spinach cooked	1/2 cup	7

Food	Serving	Fiber
Currants, black stewed with sugar		6.8
Currants, white, raw		6.8
Raisins dried		6.8
Yams (orange flesh) cooked/baked in skin	1 med (6oz)	6.8
split peas, dried	1/2 cup	6.7
Bread seven-grain	2 slices	6.5
Bread whole wheat raisin	2 slices	6.5
Flour Cornmeal (stone-ground)	1 cup	6.5
Lentils red, cooked	1 cup	6.4
Plantain boiled		6.4
Peas and carrots frozen	(5 oz.)	6.2
Bran meal	3 tbsp.	6
Bread whole wheat	2 slices	6
Cereal Bran Flakes with raisins	1 cup	6
Chickpeas (garbanzos) canned	1/2 cup	6
Noodles spinach whole wheat	1 cup	6
Spaghetti with tomato sauce	1 cup	6
Prunes (dried)	½ cup	6

Kidney beans (cooked)	½ cup	6
Peanuts, dry-roasted	½ cup	6
Lima canned or cooked	1/2 cup	5.8
Bread dark rye (whole grain)	2 slices	5.8
Currants, white stewed without sugar		5.8
Plantain green, raw		5.8
Loganberries stewed without sugar		5.7
Macaroni whole wheat, cooked	1 cup	5.7
Noodles whole wheat egg	1 cup	5.7
sweet corn canned kernels		5.7
Spaghetti whole wheat, plain	1 cup	5.6
Spaghetti with meat sauce	1 cup	5.6
Lentils brown, cooked	2/3 cup	5.5
Rice brown (before cooking)	1/2 cup	5.5
Almonds (weighed with shells)	1/4 cup	5.3
Peach stewed without sugar	1	5.3
Lemons whole	1	5.2
Loganberries stewed with sugar		5.2
Peach stewed with sugar	1	5.1

Peas and carrots boiled	1 cup	5.1
Apple baked	1 large	5
Blackberries canned, in the juice pack	1/2 cup	5
Broccoli frozen	4 spears	5
Cereal All-Bran	3 tbsp.	5
Cereal Bran Buds	3 tbsp.	5
Cereal Bran Chex	2/3 cup	5
Cereal Bran Flakes, plain	1cup	5
Cereal Raisin Bran	1 cup	5
Corn (sweet) on the cob	1 med ear	5
Corn (sweet) kernels, cooked or canned	1/2 cup	5
Corn (sweet) cream-style, canned	1/2 cup	5
Potatoes Idaho, baked	1 (7 oz.)	5
White potato, w. skin (baked)	1 medium	5
Muffins bran, whole wheat	2	4.6
Raspberries, refresh/frozen	1/2 cup	4.6
Apple raw	1 large	4.5
Artichokes cooked	I large	4.5

Artichokes canned hearts	4 or 5 sm	4.5
Blackberries raw, no sugar	1/2 cup	4.4
Shredded wheat spoon size	1 cup	4.4
Potatoes Idaho, baked	1 (6 oz.)	4.2
Yams (orange flesh) raw	1 med (6oz)	4.1
Apple raw	1 med	4
Bread Boston brown	2 slices	4
Bread pumpernickel	2 slices	4
Broccoli raw	1/2 cup	4
Cereal Cracklin' Bran	1/2 cup	4
Cereal Nabisco 100% Bran	1/2 cup	4
Cranberries sauce	1/2 cup	4
Eggplant baked with tomatoes	2 slices	4
Flour Rolled oats (whole grain)	1/3 cup	4
collards, beet greens, dandelion, kale, chard	1/2 cup	4
Mushrooms fried	1/4 cup	4
Parsnip, pared raw	1 large	4
Pear	1 med	4

Potatoes sweet: baked or boiled	1 (5 oz.)	4
Tortillas	2	4
Blueberries	1 cup	4
Pear (with peel)	1 medium	4
Quaker® Old-Fashioned Oatmeal (cooked)	1 cup	4
Leeks, raw boiled		3.9
Turnip, white tops, boiled		3.9
Yams (orange flesh) boiled	1 med (6oz)	3.9
Lima Fordhook baby, butter beans	1/2 cup	3.7
Beats whole	3 sm.	3.7
Carrots canned	1/2 cup	3.7
Lentils split, boiled	1 cup	3.7
Muffins English, whole wheat	1 whole	3.7
Mustard and watercress raw		3.7
applesauce	2/3 cup	3.6
Bread cracked wheat	2 slices	3.6
Guavas canned		3.6
Cereal Fruit N' Fiber	1/2 cup	3.5

Gooseberries ripe, raw		3.5
Potatoes boiled	1 (5 oz.)	3.5
Spinach raw	1 cup	3.5
Squash winter, baked or mashed	1/2 cup	3.5
Carrots cooked	1/2 cup	3.4
Coconut, dried sweetened	1 tbsp.	3.4
Coconut, dried unsweetened	1 tbsp.	3.4
Cornbread	1 sq. (2 1/2")	3.4
Cereal Puffed wheat	1 cup	3.3
Loganberries canned		3.3
Beans French, boiled	3/4 cup	3.2
Potatoes frozen-fried		3.2
Rutabaga (yellow turnip)	1/2 cup	3.2
beetroot raw		3.1
Beats raw	3 sm.	3.1
Cabbage, white or red savoy, raw	2/3 cup	3.1
Onion spring, raw`	3/4 cup	3.1
Sauerkraut canned	2/3 cup	3.1

Apple raw	1 small	3
Beansprouts canned		3
Banana whole	1 med 8"	3
Beans broad beans (Italian, haricot)	3/4 cup	3
Cabbage, white or red cooked	2/3 cup	3
Carrots young, boiled	1/2 cup	3
Celery, Pascal cooked	1/2 cup	3
Potatoes mashed (with 1 tbsp. milk)	1/2 cup	3
Zucchini raw or cooked	1/2 cup	3
Zucchini without sugar	1 cup	3
Tomatoes fried	1 cup	3
Apple (with peel)	1 medium	3
Banana	1 medium	3
Grapefruit	1 medium	3
Orange	1 medium	3
Sweet potato, w. skin (baked)	1 medium	3
Spinach, frozen, cooked, drained	½ cup	3
Wheat germ, toasted	2 tablespoons	3

Pear cooking raw	1 med	2.9
Rhubarb, cooked with sugar	1/2 cup	2.9
Avocado whole	1/2 avg	2.8
Parsnip, pared cooked	1 large	2.8
Watermelon	1 thick slice	2.8
Gooseberries stewed without sugar		2.7
Cereal Cornflakes	3/4 cup	2.6
Rhubarb, raw	1/2 cup	2.6
Apple baked without sugar	1 small	2.5
beetroot boiled		2.5
Beats cooked, sliced	1/2 cup	2.5
Brazil nuts shelled	2	2.5
Bread Crumbs whole wheat	1 tbsp.	2.5
Cabbage, white or red boiled	2/3 cup	2.5
Gooseberries stewed with sugar		2.5
Parsnip, pared boiled	1 large	2.5
Plums cooking, raw	2 or 3 sm	2.5
Sweet potatoes raw	1	2.5
Almonds sliced	1/4 cup	2.4

Food	Amount	Fiber
Apple cooking, raw	1 small	2.4
Orange	1 large	2.4
Rhubarb, stewed without sugar	1/2 cup	2.4
Cauliflower cooked, chopped	7/8 cup	2.3
Crackers Ry-Krisp	3	2.3
Peach raw	1 med	2.3
Pear stewed with sugar	1 med	2.3
Plums raw (weighed with pits)	2 or 3 sm	2.3
Sweet potatoes boiled	1	2.3
Crackers Wheat Thins	6	2.2
Macaroni regular, frozen with cheese, baked	10 oz.	2.2
Nectarines raw (weighed with pit)	1	2.2
Plums stewed without sugar	2 or 3 sm	2.2
Potatoes russet	1 sm	2.2
Shredded wheat large biscuit	1 piece	2.2
Zucchini raw	1/2 cup	2.2
Green (snap) beans fresh or frozen	1/2 cup	2.1
Mandarin oranges canned		2.1

Plums Victoria Dessert, raw	2 or 3 sm	2.1
Apple baked(weighed with skin)	1 small	2
Bran meal	1 tbsp.	2
Celery, Pascal raw	1/4 cup	2
Cereal Wheaties	1 cup	2
Crackers Triscuits	2	2
Cranberries raw	1/4 cup	2
Figs fresh	1	2
Mushrooms canned sliced, water-pack	1/4 cup	2
Plums	2 or 3 sm	2
Rice white (before cooking)	1/2 cup	2
Squash summer (yellow)	1/2 cup	2
Turnip, white cooked	1/2 cup	2
Pineapple	1 cup	2
Asparagus (5 medium, cooked)	½ cup	2
Broccoli (cooked)	½ cup	2
Carrots	½ cup	2
Cauliflower (cooked)	½ cup	2
Rye bread	1 slice	2

Whole-wheat bread	1 slice	2
Brown rice, cooked	½ cup	2
Spaghetti, cooked	1 cup	2
Apple stewed with sugar	1 small	1.9
Bread white	2 slices	1.9
Chestnuts roasted	2 lg	1.9
Plums stewed with sugar	2 or 3 sm	1.9
Prunes pitted	3	1.9
Tangerines raw	1	1.9
Apricots stewed without sugar	1 small	1.7
Asparagus cooked, small spears	1/2 cup	1.7
Avocado diced	1/4 cup	1.7
Carrots raw, slivered (4-5 sticks)	1/4 cup	1.7
Cherries cooking, raw	10	1.7
Mulberries raw		1.7
Pear eating(weighed with skin and core)	1med	1.7
Pear canned		1.7
Flour All-purpose (white)	1 cup	1.6

Okra fresh or frozen, cooked	1/2 cup	1.6
Apple eating (weighed with skin & core)	1 small	1.5
Cabbage, white or red raw	1/2 cup	1.5
Honeydew melon	3" slice	1.5
Lettuce raw	1	1.5
Mangoes raw	1	1.5
Onion cooked	1/2 cup	1.5
Orange raw (weighed with peel and pits)	1sm	1.5
Peanut butter homemade	1 tbsp.	1.5
Cherries stewed without sugar	10	1.4
Crackers Graham	2	1.4
Mushrooms raw	5 sm	1.4
Parsnip, pared	1 sm	1.4
Peach canned in light syrup	2 halves	1.4
Tomatoes raw	1 sm.	1.4
Apricots canned		1.3
Tangerines raw(with peel and seeds)	1	1.3
Cauliflower raw, chopped	3 buds	1.2

Cherries sweet, raw	10	1.2
Cherries stewed with sugar	10	1.2
Dates, pitted	2 (1/2 oz.)	1.2
Olives green	6	1.2
Olives black	6	1.2
Orange	1 sm	1.2
Peppers green sweet, cooked	1/2 cup	1.2
Peppers red chili, fresh	1 tbsp.	1.2
Peppers dried, crushed	1 tsp.	1.2
Turnip, white raw, slivered	1/4 cup	1.2
Fruit pie filling canned		1.1
Fruit salad canned		1.1
Peanut butter	1 tbsp.	1.1
Peanuts dry roasted	1 tbsp.	1.1
Walnuts English, shelled, chopped	1 tbsp.	1.1
Cantaloupe	4 pieces	1
Celery, Pascal chopped	2 tbsp.	1
Grapes white	20	1
Grapes red or black	15-20	1

Mangoes canned		1
Peach canned		1
Peppers red sweet (pimento)	2 tbsp.	1
Popcorn (no oil, butter or margarine)	1 cup	1
Potatoes boiled		1
Radishes	1 tbsp.	1
Raspberry jam	1 tbsp.	1
Zucchini canned		1
Tomatoes canned	1/2 cup	1
Watercress raw	1/2 cup	1
Cantaloupe	1 cup	1
Tomato	1 medium	1
White bread	1 slice	1
Avocado sliced	2 slices	0.9
Melons, cantaloupe yellow, honeydew, raw	3 slices	0.9
Bean sprouts raw in salad	1/4 cup	0.8
Grapefruit	1/2 avg	0.8
(Boston, leaf, iceberg) shredded lettuce	1 cup	0.8

Onion green, raw (scallion)	1/4 cup	0.8
Pineapple fresh, cubed	1/2 cup	0.8
Pineapple canned	1 cup	0.8
Blackberries jam, with seeds	1 tbsp.	0.7
Cucumber, raw unpeeled	10 slices	0.7
Rice instant	1 serving	0.7
Almonds slivered	1 tbsp.	0.6
Endive, raw salad	10 leaves	0.6
Parsley, chopped	2 tbsp.	0.6
cranberry-orange relish	1 tbsp.	0.5
lychees raw		0.5
Pumpkin raw		0.5
Sunflower kernels	1 tbsp.	0.5
relish	1 tbsp.	0.5
Tomatoes sauce	1/2 cup	0.5
Gooseberries canned		0.4
lychees canned		0.4
Onion instant minced	1 tbsp.	0.3
Parsley, chopped	1 tbsp.	0.3

Peppers green sweet, raw	2 tbsp.	0.3
White rice, cooked	½ cup	0.3
Onion raw	1 tbsp.	0.2
Tomatoes catsup	1 tbsp.	0.2
Flour All-purpose (white)	1 tbsp.	0.1
Flour Cornstarch	1 tbsp.	0.1
Radishes	3	0.1
Lemons juice, fresh	1 glass	0
Orange juice, fresh	1 glass	0

As you can see from this chart, the following foods are great fiber food to add to your diet if you have not yet done so.

5: What to Eat for Breakfast

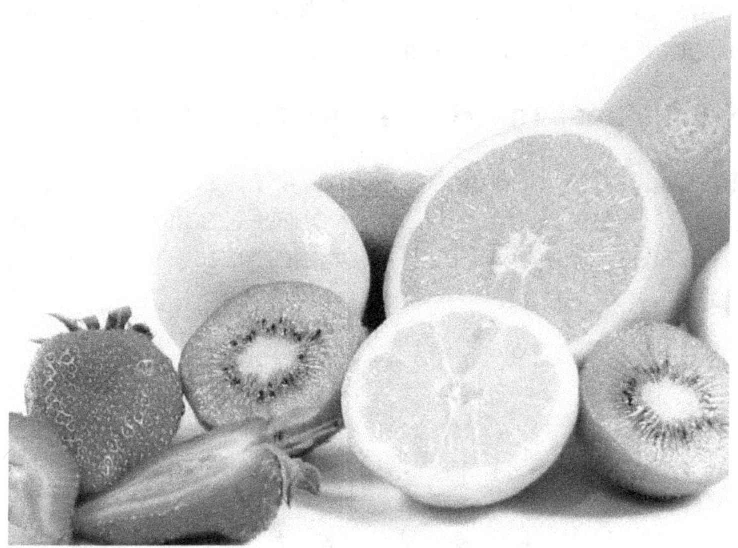

Morning Time

Morning is the time to load up on fruits, fruit juices, vegetable juices, teas, tonics, or special nutritional drinks.

From early morning to noon is the time your body is releasing toxins and excess nutrients it no longer needs. During your sleep, your body was busy removing toxins and unwanted material from your cells, tissues, and organs. It brings this excess waste material into your bladder and colon

Your body needs to expel these wastes after you wake up. This is the detoxifying process your body goes through every morning until noon.

You can create great health by helping your body cleanse and detoxify properly. You do this by only eating and drinking those foods that promote urine and bowels movements. You need to eat this way from the time you wake and until noon time.

Fruits and various drinks promote waste elimination by allowing your body to concentrate on this process. Fruits and liquids are digested within 1 to 2 hours and put pressure on your bladder and colon to eliminate.

Heavy Breakfast Interferes with Detoxification

If you eat a heavy breakfast like, eggs, bread, butter, potatoes, bacon, meat, or other solid protein and carbohydrates, you will block your morning body detoxification process.

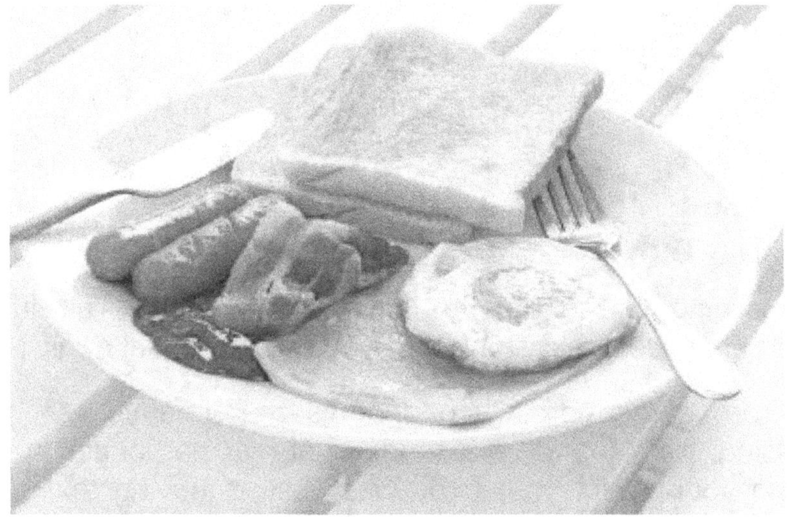

A heavy breakfast takes a good 3 to 5 hours to digest. This digestion causes your body to concentrate on digesting the heavy meal instead of concentration on detoxification.

Morning Drinks

When you first get up in the morning, drink some liquid like a lemon drink, green tea, water with a slight amount of juice, or a chlorophyll drink. This will help to cleanse out your esophagus down to your colon.

Chlorophyll Drink

You can make a chlorophyll drink by buying liquid chlorophyll. Add 1-2 tablespoons, more if you like, of chlorophyll into 8 oz. of water. Squeeze the juice of one lemon into the water. The lemon juice will help to make this drink more palatable.

Another morning drink that prepares you for the morning is a combination of orange, grapefruit, and lemon. Use a manual fruit extractor to create juices. You can add a bit of water or honey if the juice is too thick or tart.

After a quick liquid drink, you can start eating fruit or drinking a fruit smoothie.

Strawberry lemonade

Add to 6-8 oz. of water some strawberries. Now add the insides of one small lemon, using a spoon to pull out the juice and pulp. Throw this into a blender with a bit of honey, and blend at low speed for one minute.

Instead of using strawberries, you can use a mango and lemon or lime. In a blender combine them with some honey. Add some water to make it the consistency you like. Without water, you can consider this a pudding and eat it with a spoon.

Morning Fruit bowl

At the beginning of this program, choose those fruits, for your fruit bowl, that contain the most fiber. Later, you can use fruits that have less fiber, so that you can get the benefits of these fiber foods.

Make a list of the fruits to eat in the morning and buy them for coming days from the farmers market. Try to get those fruits that are organic or have very little pesticide spraying.

Include many seasonal fruits such as:

Apples, Apricots, Avocados, Bananas, Blueberries, Boysenberries, Cantaloupes, Cherries, Figs, Dates, raw or dried, Strawberries, peaches, Dried prunes,

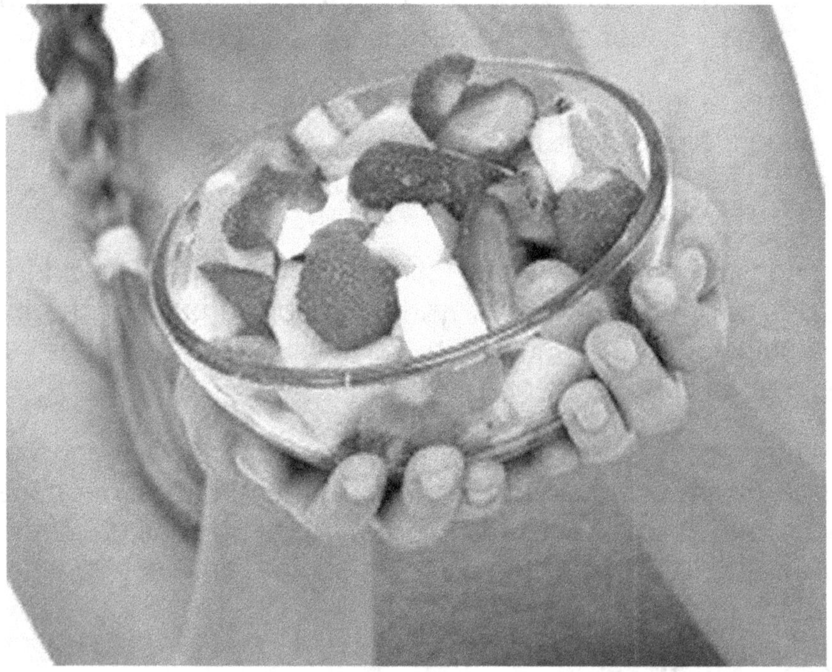

This fruit bowl will help your detoxification morning and start your fiber day.

Smoothies

If you prefer drinking a smoothie, here is how you can get started. Making a smoothie that gives you a high fiber count and morning energy is easy. Once you get used to making it, you will find it hard not to start your day without it.

Smoothie for the day

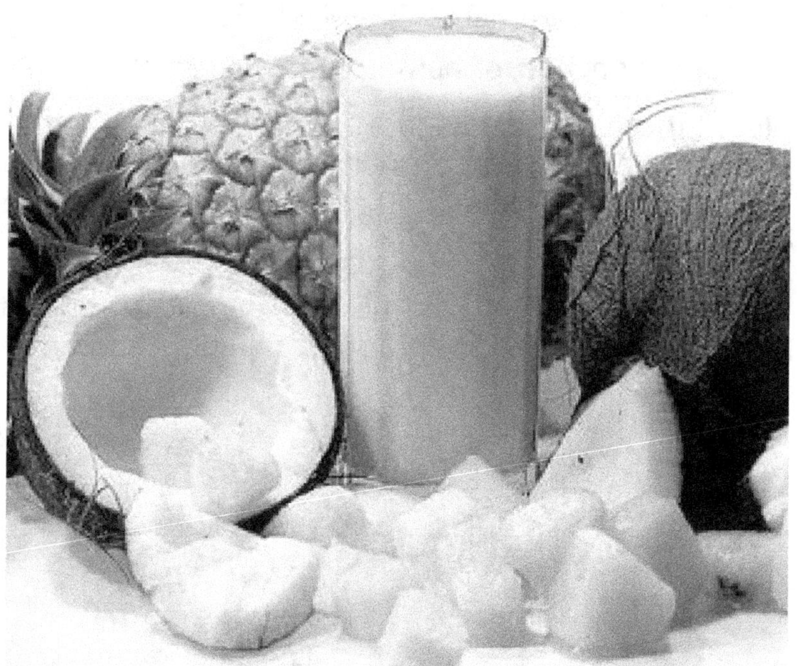

Here is a list of smoothie ingredients that you can use as a base for all the smoothies you make.

- Liquid base: 8 oz. or more of any 100% juice without sugar, almond milk, or just plain water.

- 2 bananas – to thicken the smoothie

- ½ cup of fresh papaya to help digestion

- ½ cup of fresh pineapple or any other fruit that you prefer

- 1 heaping teaspoon of oat or rice bran for fiber

- One teaspoon of coconut oil for short chain fatty acids (SCFA)

- One teaspoon chia seed for energy

- One teaspoon of lemon for minerals

- A drop of honey for nutrients and good taste

Mix all these ingredients in a blender for up to 2 minutes under low power to prevent heating up the mixture. You can add a couple of ice cube so that you can blend at a high power.

Use these ingredients as the base, and then add other fruits of your choice. You can also at this time add any high protein, green, or fruit powder.

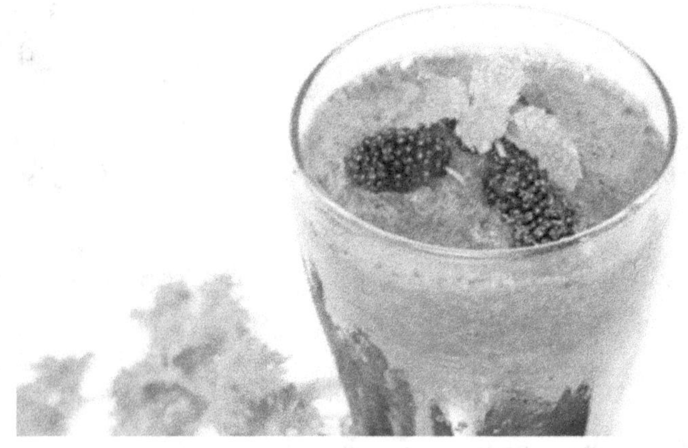

Experiment with your smoothie until you get the taste, and consistency you want.

Mixed Strawberry Berry Smoothie

Here is a quick smoothie that you can make if you are in a hurry.

Put the following berries into your blender:

- Blueberries, strawberries, blackberries, or another type of berry that you have
- Goat yogurt or sugar-free yogurt
- Add a bit of honey if it needed

If you want to cool this smoothie, add a couple of ice cubes

Pineapple Mango Smoothie

- Add the following to a blender:
- Fresh pineapple chunks
- Fresh mango chunks
- One or small two bananas or one large one
- Juice of one lime or lemon
- Honey to sweeten
- Water or 100% apple juice or any other juice that you have.

In all the above recipes you can use 100% juice of any flavor that you like.

6: What to Eat for Lunch or Dinner

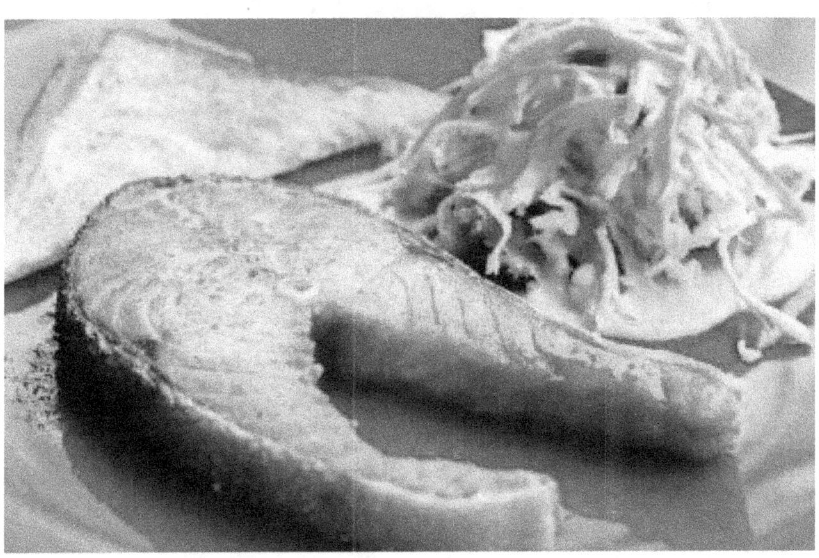

Main Meals

At lunch or dinner, it's time to add more fiber to your diet. At this time, you can have a heavy meal, which includes meat, fish, or carbohydrates. But, by including a nice salad, you can add more fiber for the day, and in addition, this will help you digest your food better.

Without eat a fresh vegetable salad at this time, you will be prone to constipation.

Meat and process carbohydrates don't have fiber. A lunch salad is necessary to provide fiber that will later combine with your digested meat waste in your colon. This will reduce the amount of time that this waste remains in your colon.

So here are some typical lunch menus.

- Salad

- Beef, chicken, pork

- fish

- Legumes

- Carbohydrates

Deserts after Meals

Avoid sugar deserts, fruits after lunch. Also, try to avoid sodas or other drinks with sugar. Minimize the amount of water you drink with your meal. Water dilutes your stomach acids, which makes it more difficult for you to digest your food properly.

What you eat for lunch is sometimes dictated by the restaurant that you go to. If this is the case, a good serving of meat, carbohydrates or sandwich, with a salad is fine.

If you eat pasta of any kind eat it with a salad

If you eat a sandwich make sure it contains lettuce with other vegetables.

If you don't like salads, try sprinkling it with raisins to see if it makes more desirable.

If you are home then, you have more flexibility as what you eat for lunch or dinner. There many protein or carbohydrate recipes that you can cook. Just always include a salad with your main dish.

It is always best to eat your salad first before your main meal.

Fish and salad are an excellent lunch.

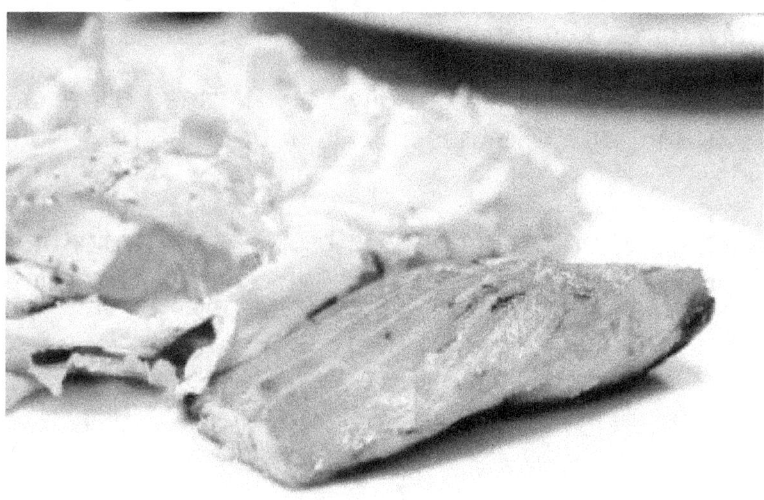

Meat and salad

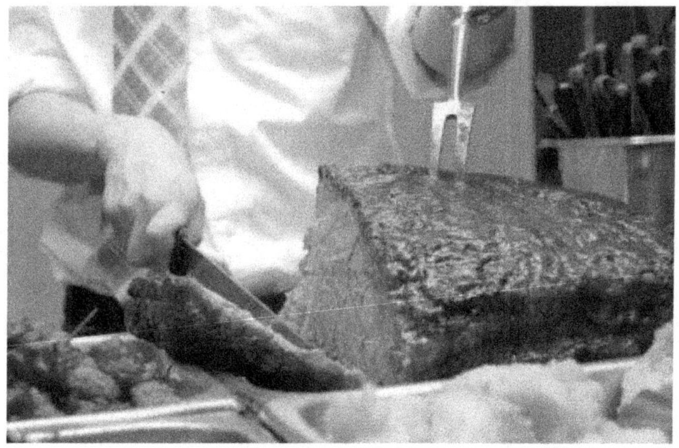

Just add a salad for this lunch meat.

Here are some other ideas

- Beans and salad

- Eggs and salad

- Chicken or beef burrito

- Carbohydrates and salad

Minimize eating meat that is high in saturated fat.

Get your good fat from olive oil, flaxseed oil, avocado oil, and coconut oil. Use these oils in your smoothies, soups, and salads.

On occasion, you can eat butter, but avoid margarine. Margarine contains triglycerides, which creates cardiovascular problems.

7: Final Thoughts on Fiber

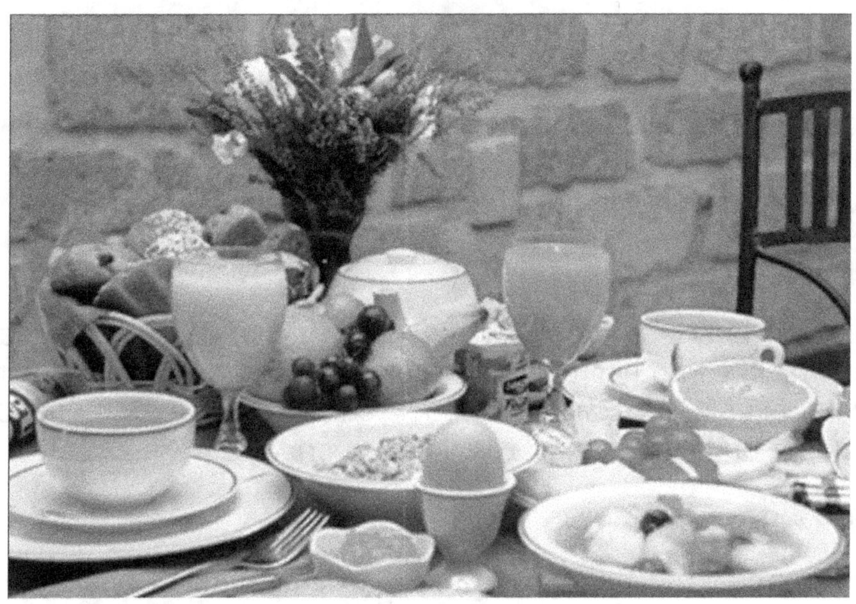

Morning Drink

Use a morning drink every day. If you drink green tea before your fruits, you will have less body inflammation. Green tea is high an anti-inflammatory chemical. It is excellent for cardiovascular issue, problems, or diseases. It also will help with prostate problems.

Add apples to your fruit bowl every day for constipation. Any type of apple you eat is ok, but gala or Fuji apples are good since some are small and crisp.

It is best to use fresh organic apples and fruits. Inorganic fruits have been sprayed with a variety of chemicals that you are unaware of. If apples are not organic, it is better to peel the apple before eating.

High Fiber Foods

High fiber foods include bran, broccoli, cabbage, berries, leafy greens, celery, squash, beans, mushrooms, figs, and dried fruit.

Any increase in fiber that you eat will benefit your health. You may never be eating 30 or 45 grams of fiber every day. This number is just a reference number, which represents an average consumption of fiber you should strive for.

Daily Fiber Count

You may only need 25 mg of fiber per day to get good health, but another person may need 30 mg. But, for sure most people are short on fiber based on the tremendous amount of illnesses that exist in the world.

Use Fiber Charts

Look at the fiber food values to start adding fiber foods that you have not yet used. Within a few months, you will not need to check fiber values. Eating the right amount of fiber will become natural to you.

8: Author & Resources

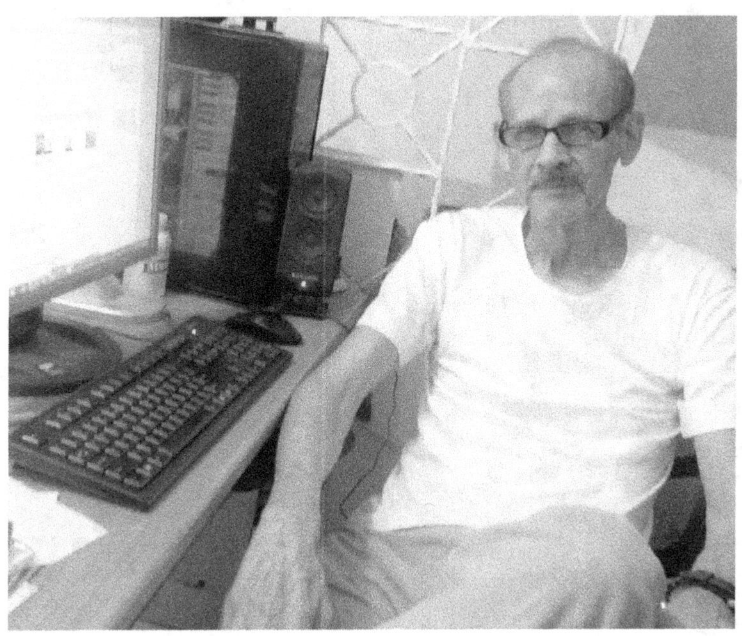

Nutritional Consultant

Rudy Silva is a natural nutritional consultant educated in the United State of Nutrition and Physics. He is a graduate of San Jose State University in California. He is the author of 45 other e-books and physical books on natural diets for various illnesses. He has authored a newsletter in natural remedies for over 4 years.

If you need support or want to promote any of his e-books, please contact him at rss41@yahoo.com and expect a reply within 24 hours.   He looks forward to hearing from you and is happy to help you understand his material on natural and nutritional health.

Give a Review

And, don't forget to give a review for this book, so that others can gain the benefits of what is in this book. A review can be just a few sentences.

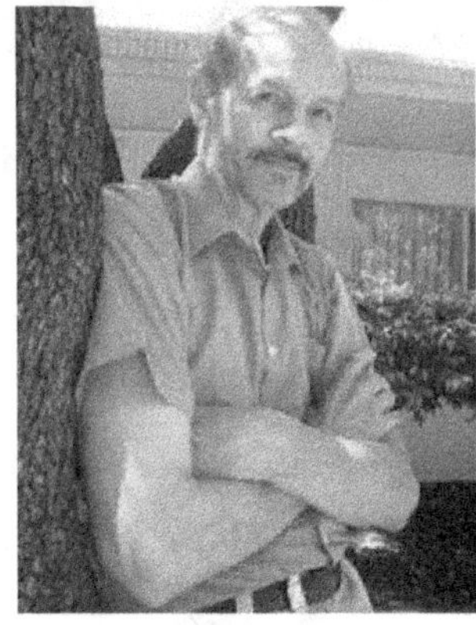

Rudy S. Silva, Natural Nutritionist

www.ingramcontent.com/pod-product-compliance
Lightning Source LLC
Chambersburg PA
CBHW070051260726
48658CB00002B/834